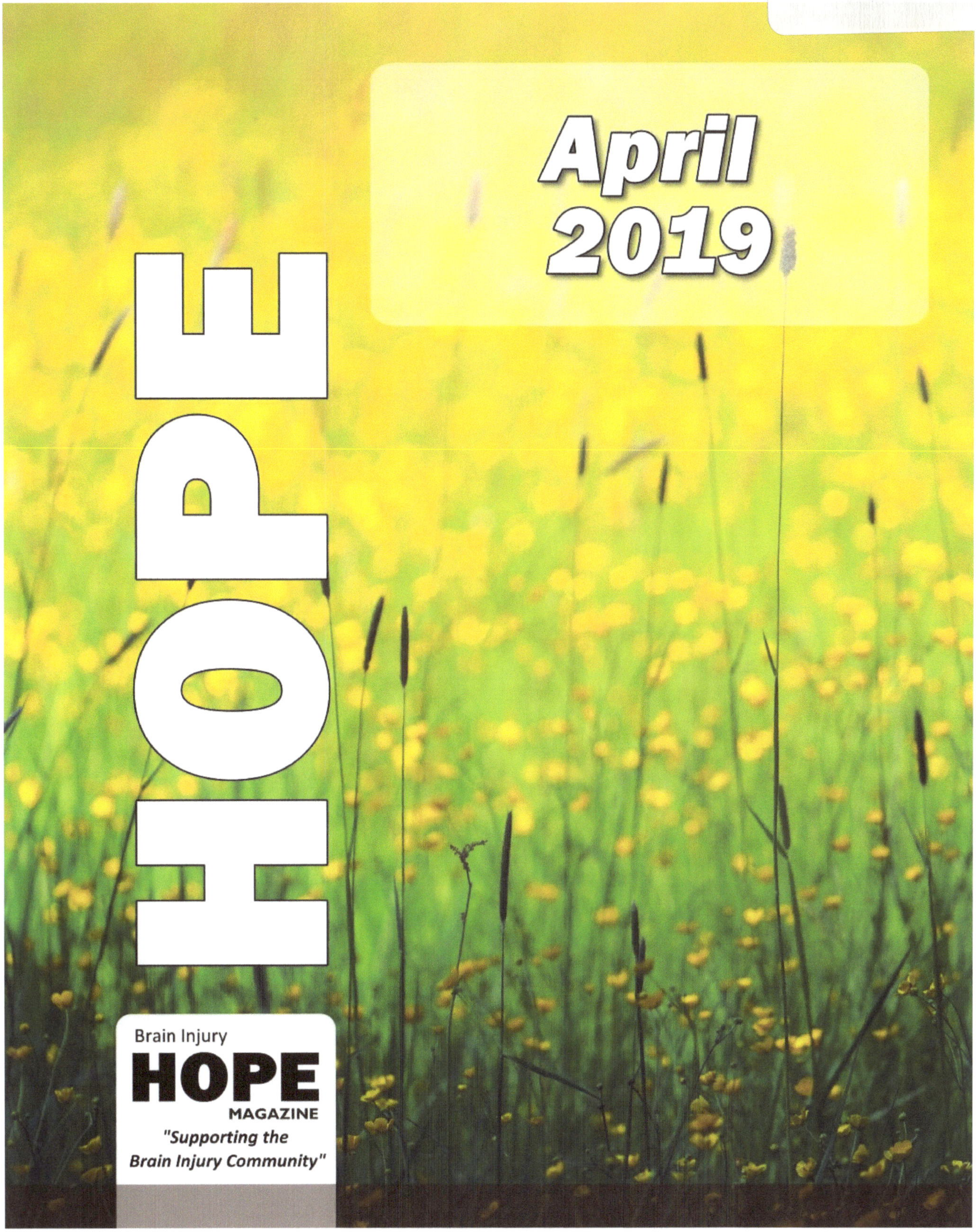

April 2019

HOPE

Brain Injury
HOPE
MAGAZINE
"Supporting the Brain Injury Community"

Welcome

HOPE MAGAZINE

Serving the Brain Injury Community

April 2019

Publisher
David A. Grant

Editor
Sarah Grant

Our Contributors

Tobie-Lynn Andrade
Michelle Bartlett
Nicole Bingaman
David A. Grant
Kiana Kay
Kelly Lang
Abby Maslin
Tracie Massie
Jeff Willis

Welcome to the April 2019 issue of HOPE Magazine

Amazingly, this is the first issue of our fifth consecutive year of publication. We are welcoming year five with an amazing array of contributing writers.

Included in this month's issue are stories from survivors, family members, as well as caregivers.

One of the great joys of our journey is to feel the excitement when we reach out to a contributor to let them know that we will be publishing their story to a worldwide readership. Their spirits are bolstered with the profound realization that they do indeed have the ability to serve others, and that the toughest experience of their lives can serve a greater good.

It is our hope that you come away from this month's issue with a renewed spirit, and of course a new hope. In the final analysis, that is what we strive for – to offer real hope to those who need it most.

Peace,

David A. Grant
Publisher

Contents

Make a habit of two things: to help, or at least to do no harm.

-Hippocrates

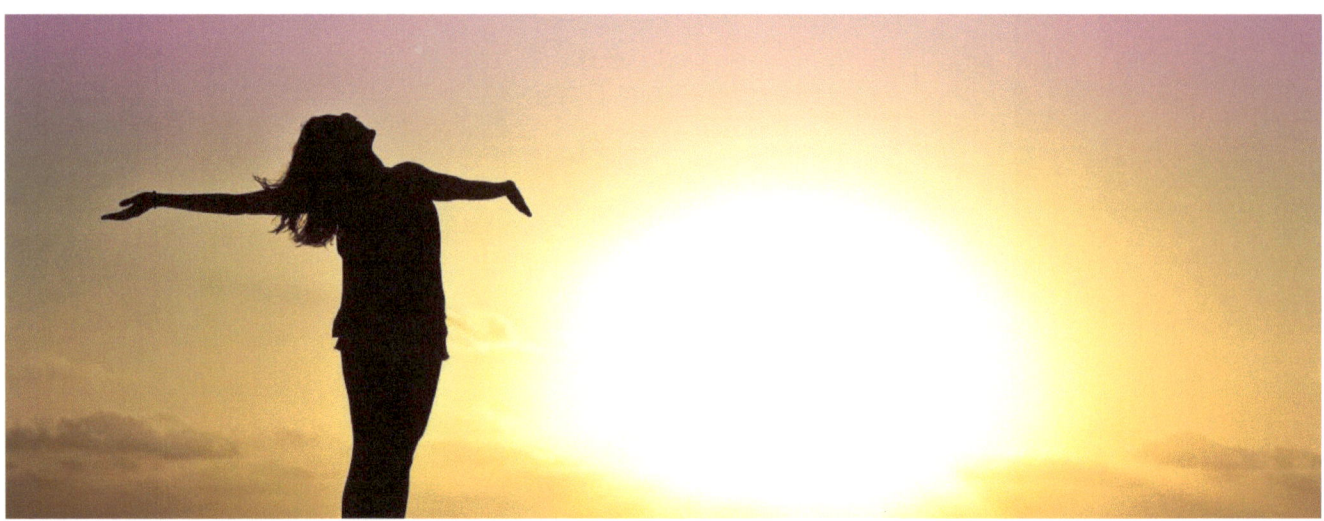

Year Fifteen

By Michelle Bartlett

As I sit here and write this fifteen years after my severe anoxic brain injury, in March of 2004, I am amazed at how far I have advanced. I could've never imagined what the future had in store for me.

I remember the day I went for open heart surgery – all too well, actually. The vivid memories still remain to this day. I remember being scared out of my mind but trying to be strong for my family. The pain when I woke up from the surgery was unimaginable.

Then, there is nothing. Absolutely nothing!

Two days after the surgery I went into complete cardiac

> "The decision was made to remove life support and move me to palliative care. My organs had begun to fail."

and pulmonary arrest. There was no oxygen to my brain for seven to ten minutes. It took the doctors hours to stabilize me, but I was pronounced brain dead with no hope of survival. My family refused to give up until I developed pneumonia. The decision was made to remove life support and move me to palliative care. My organs had begun to fail.

One day in palliative care, my long-time best friend was brushing my hair and I said "ouch." Quickly, I was transferred back to the neurological wing. Tests were run and my brain scans showed activity. I can't even begin to imagine how relieved they must have felt.

"I knew something bad had happened. I didn't understand what or how it would impact the rest of my life."

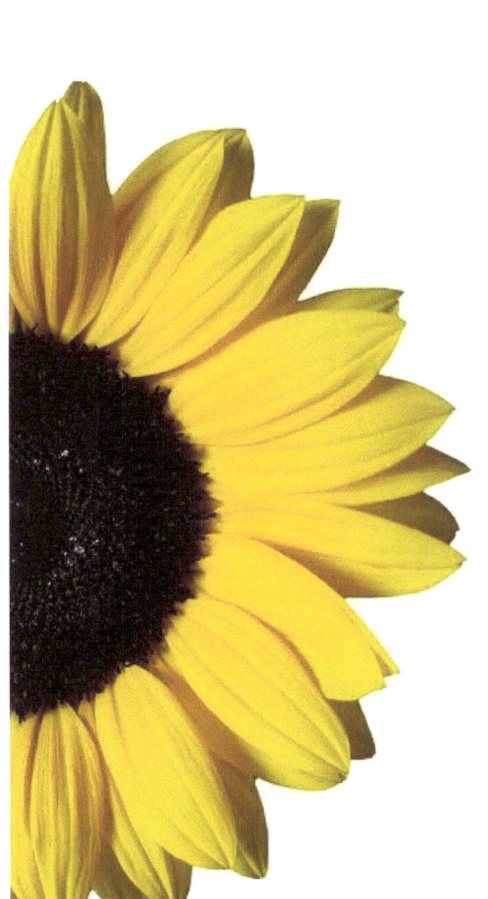

In the beginning, I was like a baby needing help with anything and everything. My vision was limited at best. My memory was non-existent. I slept all the time, literally. It was this bone weary, brain weary, total exhaustion I had never experienced before. I could not hold a conversation with people and would quickly lose track of what we were talking about. Loud noises and bright lights were terrifying. I had no sense of time or space. If left alone I got lost easily.

I knew something bad had happened. I didn't understand what or how it would impact the rest of my life.

The first year I made huge improvements and we were told by the medical professionals that I had reached the upper limits of my recovery. That wasn't good enough for me. I didn't know what I wanted but I knew it was more than what I had.

There was a deep-seated will in me not only to survive but to thrive.

I know the old saying "hindsight is 20/20" is true, as I look back on the last fifteen years. I knew who I wanted to be. I wanted to be the "old Michelle." I saw her reflection in the mirror everyday but inside Michelle had been replaced with someone else. She was someone I didn't know. That in itself was frightening and very confusing.

Looking back now, I had no idea what I was doing. I needed to do something, anything, to improve. How I wished for "that magic wand," that could fix my brain. I was miserable not being able to function at a level I thought I should. It was a constant internal battle within myself. I refused to accept the "permanently disabled; never to work again" label. Acceptance was a term I had yet to fully understand. I felt like I had no value, no voice as a person; I was a throw-away; a burden to society. My self-esteem and confidence had been utterly shattered.

All the dreams I had for a "normal" life, I thought, were gone. Children, marriage, travel, and a career would never happen to a disabled injured woman.

There were days that the mountain seemed too impossible to climb; too confusing. I got lost.

I knew what the problem "was" – I was broken but I didn't know how to "fix" it or what steps to take to "fix" me.

A brain injury can't be fixed. There is no "magic pill." That is where I got stuck in my desperation for survival.

It took many years and many hours of hard and exhausting work before I was able to have dreams and goals for the future again.

I do now – BIG ones.

Living independently, travelling, public speaking; even something as small as being able to pay my own bills I can do now, and so much more. All the things that I had been told all those years ago I could never do again.

Am I proud of who I am now? YOU BET! I am a survivor! Do I have a bright future now? YES!

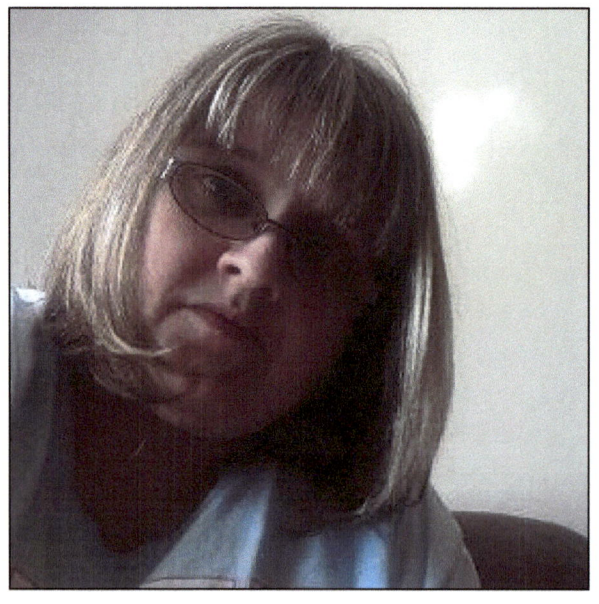

Meet Michelle Bartlett

Michelle survived a severe anoxic brain injury two days after open-heart surgery in March of 2004. She has made a remarkable recovery. In 2016, Michelle was awarded the Volunteer Award of Merit from Brain Injury Canada. Then, in the fall of 2018, she was awarded the prestigious Debbie and Trevor Greene Award of Courage for her extraordinary heroic contribution to the cause of acquired brain injury in Canada from Brain Injury Canada. She has lived all across Canada and loves to travel. Michelle supports and advocates for brain injury survivors in Canada and manages numerous groups. Currently Michelle resides in New Brunswick Canada.

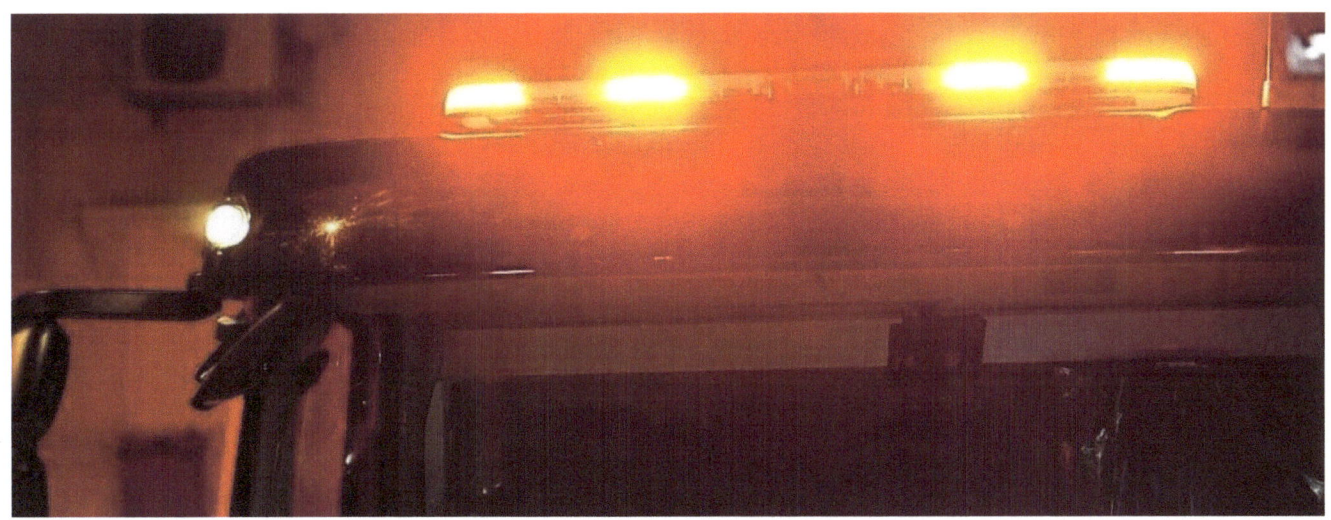

Our Superheroes

By Kelly Lang

Every year on the anniversary of our horrific accident my husband Mike and I have tried to honor the local Rescue Squad who responded. These men and women are the true heroes. They are the ones who sometimes risk their lives to help others. They saved our daughter's life on November 27, 2001.

We have asked ourselves two questions over and over the past 17 years. How do you thank the people who saved your child's life and who were the individuals involved at that moment? We discovered the answer to the second question a few weeks ago.

Every year we visit our local Rescue Squad and drop off a note of thanks and a few gifts. Once Olivia learned about the fateful day she wanted to write the note herself and made sure we went on the anniversary of the accident, or as close to the date as possible. Some years it was difficult to find a time when someone would be in the building to accept the gift. I recall one such incident when we stopped by four times before someone answered the buzzer.

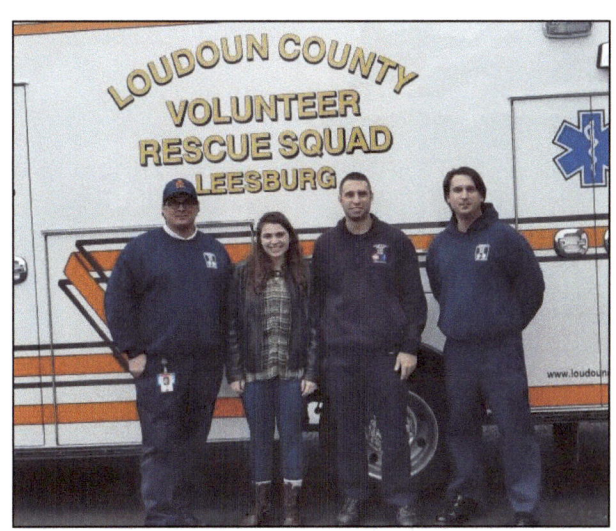

This year the anniversary fell on a Tuesday. Mike would be at work and our youngest daughter, Anya, would be at school. Olivia and I set out to take care of the gift.

In all honesty, I had taken a step back from going. It is difficult. So many memories come flooding back. As with many things in life I knew I had to be brave for her so I forged ahead. Luckily, there were three emergency medical technicians in the building when we arrived. Olivia handed them her homemade card and I presented the gift baskets. The gentlemen were very welcoming and asked her some questions. I asked if I could take pictures and they enthusiastically agreed. We stepped outside and they stood in front of one of their trucks for better lighting. The Chief asked for an email address, in case he wrote something for their newsletter, and I gave him mine.

We expressed our gratitude one more time and headed on our way to lunch and manicures. Over the last few years, I have tried to make this day more of a celebration rather than a day of mourning. Yes, it is still a sad day for me but I was trying to turn the intention around.

The following day I received an email that shocked me. It was from another Battalion Chief who saw the thank you note while at a meeting.

He thought the story sounded familiar and wondered if we were involved in a rescue call that haunted him all these years. I responded with more details and he confirmed he and his partner had been the first to arrive on the scene and they worked to save my girl.

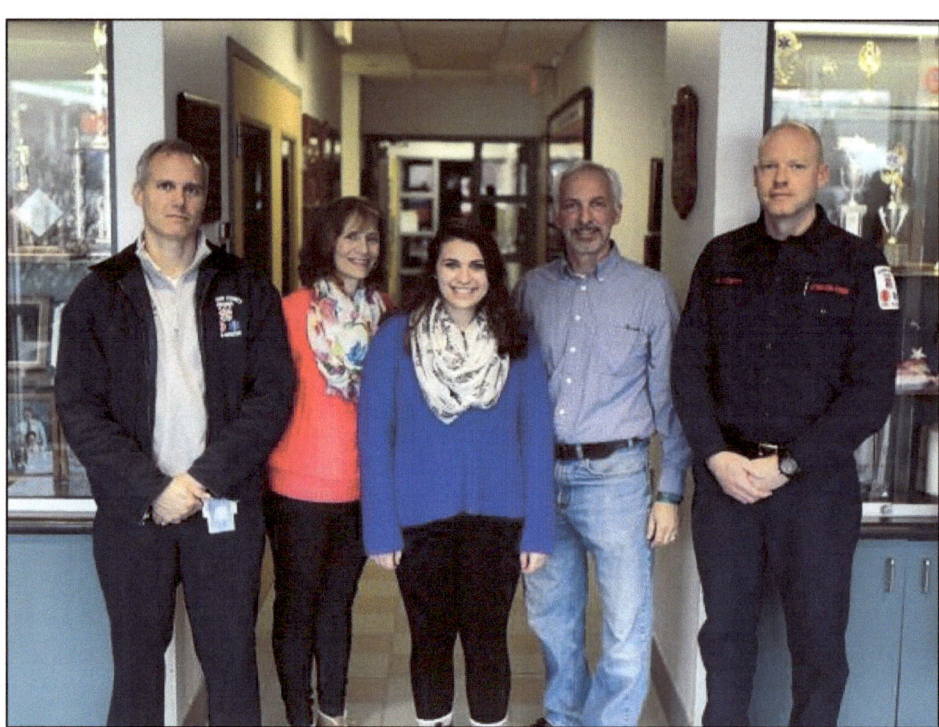

We spoke a few days later and he relayed the story of her rescue, after I told him I didn't remember much about the accident. He explained that when he approached the vehicle he thought she was sleeping and thought it was strange. It wasn't until he put his hand on her chest that he realized she wasn't breathing. The car door wouldn't open so he pulled her out along with the car seat through the already broken window.

She was brought to the ambulance where they tried to get her breathing while immediately transporting her to the local emergency room. The details he remembered were unbelievable. He told me the memory of some calls is forgotten for various reasons but this was one that stayed with him over the years.

Mike, Olivia, and I arranged to meet him and his partner. I was a nervous wreck beforehand. I don't know why. After all, how do you thank the two men who saved your child's life? We contacted a local newspaper beforehand and asked if they wanted a "feel good" story. Surprisingly, our story appeared on the front page of our county newspaper and a local radio station interviewed me and ran a story the following day.

We were thrilled to finally meet our two heroes and tell them how grateful we were for all they have done for our family. As expected, they were very humble. I still don't feel we can ever thank them enough. How do you thank someone for saving a life?

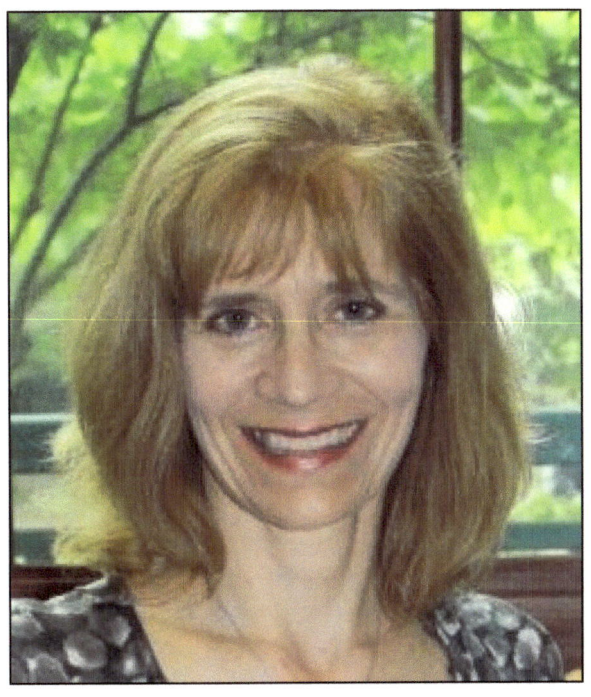

Meet Kelly Lang

Kelly Lang is a brain injury survivor and caregiver to her daughter, Olivia, who sustained a traumatic brain injury in 2001, at the age of 3. Kelly lives in Leesburg, Virginia with her husband Michael, daughters Hannah (22), Olivia (20), and Anya (10).

Kelly is a board member of the Brain Injury Association of Virginia, a member of the Brain Injury Association of America Brain Injury Council, a peer visitor at Fairfax Hospital and a speaker for Brain Injury Services, Inc.

Kelly and her husband created a website, www.themiraclechild.org, to educate others about brain injury.

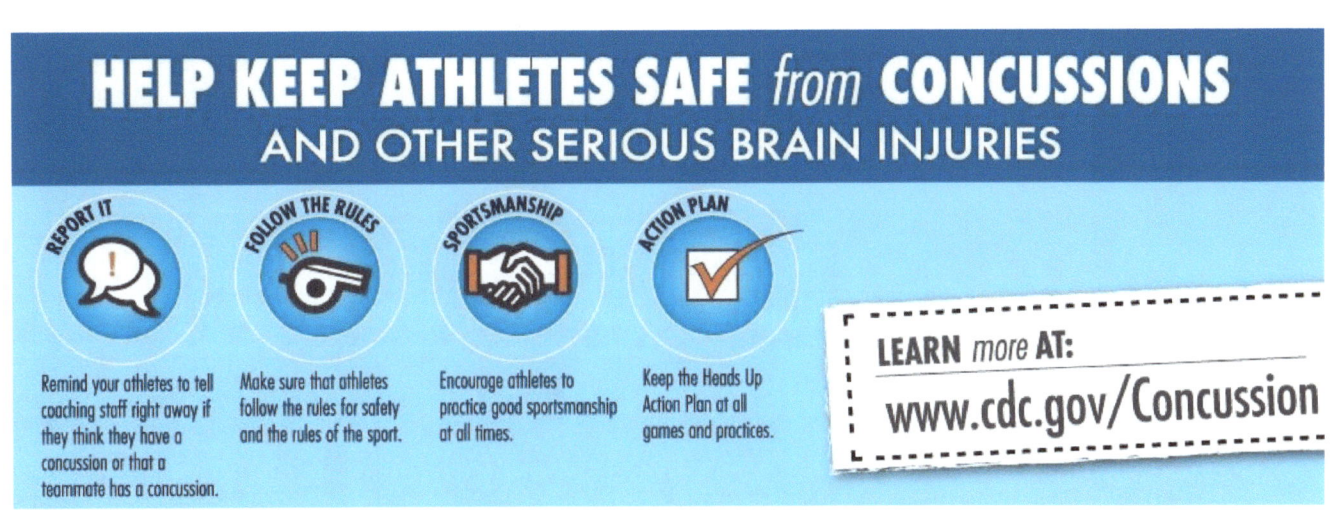

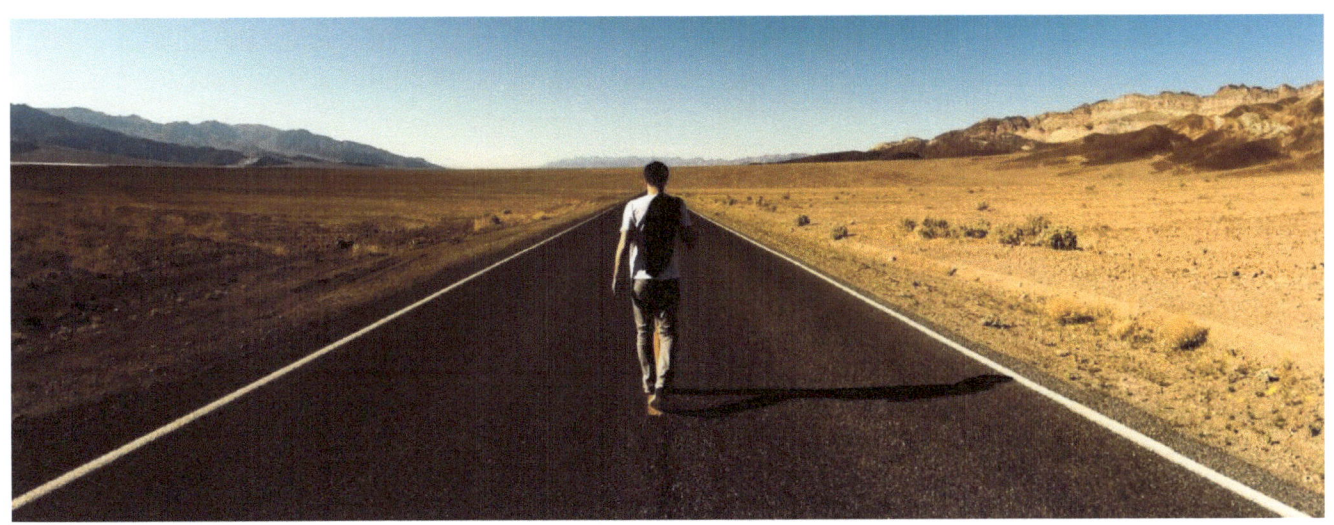

My TBI Journey
By Jeff Willis

I never would have guessed it would happen to me. By "it" I mean four strokes and an aneurysm all at once. I lived an amazing life as an industrial painter. I took pride in my work and came home to my beautiful red-headed wife and three children each day. I was a father, husband, son, coworker, and provider. On New Year's Day in 2006, the life I knew turned upside down. "New Year's" is certainly about change. That change in my life meant learning how to do essentially everything all over again.

I don't remember much, but from what I am told I suddenly had an onset of bizarre symptoms while working on my Dodge Dakota in the driveway at my house in Colorado. My wife Cherie knew something was wrong. I was transported to North Suburban medical hospital where everyone learned I had four strokes and an aneurysm, then was flown on flight for life to Swedish hospital.

> "I was transported to North Suburban medical hospital where everyone learned I had four strokes and an aneurysm."

My wife was told there was little chance of my survival and in the case that I did survive, my quality of life would be compared to a "vegetable." My mother passed down a hereditary stroke disorder called CADASIL syndrome that made me susceptible to this kind of injury. However, I never imagined I would go through something like this. I also never knew exactly what a brain injury was. If you would have told me that I would have this severe of an injury and survived it years ago, I would have never believed you.

After being admitted to Swedish hospital, I was on life support for a month in the intensive care unit. Over the next several years I had to again learn how to walk, talk, read, write, communicate, eat, swallow, and everything in between. I felt completely lost and admittedly don't remember much of my recovery for the first four-to-five years.

There were stages I went through in this time that were difficult and strange. Some of the stages included hallucinations, food and drinks exhibiting a "mud-like" taste, a feeling of constant motion as if being on a moving bus, balance and coordination problems that made me walk on my tippy-toes, stunted hair-growth, agnosia (being unable to correctly identify objects), disorientation (being unable to detect time and space), and a disrupted sleep schedule. However, in that time I made huge strides such as getting out of my wheelchair, remembering family and friends again, being able to hold a conversation, and many other things.

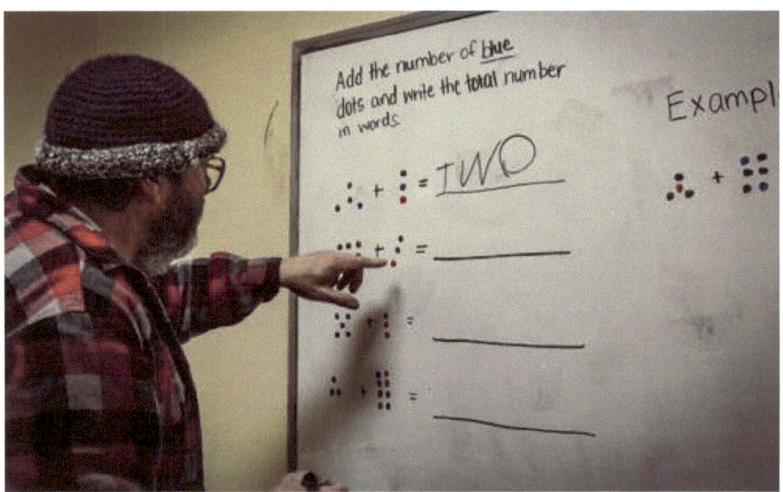

I am still working on learning basic skills each and every day such as improving my memory, learning how to socialize appropriately, navigating the grocery store, decreasing impulsive behaviors, etc. What has helped me the most has been God, my family, independent living skills trainers, Dr. Guri Singh (my primary care doctor), and a day program. You really have to get to a point where you can accept help from everyone. This doesn't take away from your unique abilities and attributes. You still have so much to give to the world and other survivors. Since I have been so accepting of care and advice, here's mine to all of you who have sustained a TBI:

- Give it to God
- Interact and make connections with other brain injury survivors – we can help one another
- Never stop sharing your story
- Pick up hobbies that keep your mind occupied, such as fishing
- Stay humorous, tell jokes and never take life too seriously
- Ask loved ones and caregivers to remind you of your progress
- Stay proactive with your health
- Always have goals to accomplish
- Exercise at least one time per week
- Challenge yourself to cognitive activities
- Have something to take care of such as a plant, an animal, etc.
- Get some sunshine
- Remember: the brain is an amazing organ, don't underestimate its ability to grow

Brain injuries come in many forms. Regardless of the cause, we all experience loss and changes. You can't change the circumstance, but you can change your attitude. Brain injuries are hard to describe, but I like to think of them as a chance for a new life, a time to start over.

When life is slowed down you learn to love deeper, find inventive ways to do things, and find beauty in the details. "Life is like a box of chocolates, you never know what you're going to get" -Forrest Gump. Sometimes your chocolate is a brain injury.

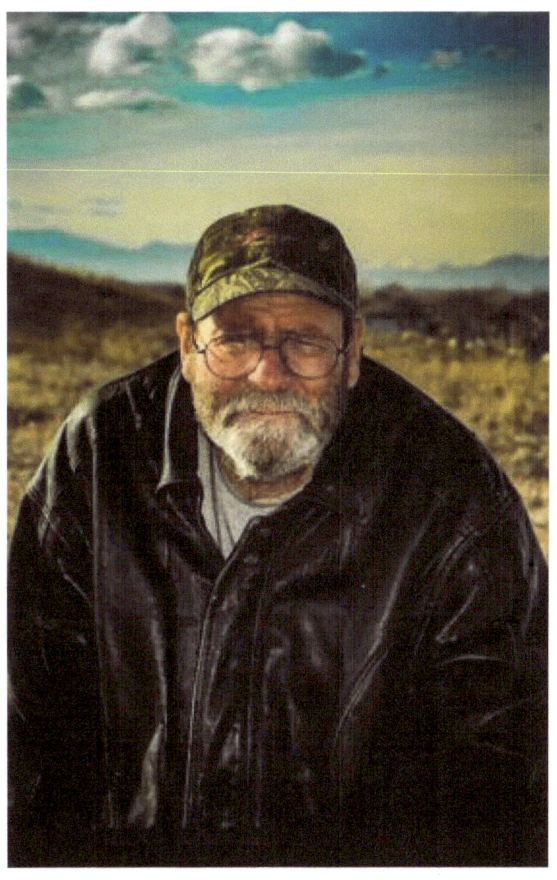

Meet Jeff Willis

Jeff Willis is 60 years old and was born in Pineville, Louisiana. Throughout his life he has lived in several states including Louisiana, Texas, Georgia, and Colorado (where he currently resides). He has worked several jobs including fishing on an oyster boat, selling car parts for Chevrolet, and painting for an industrial painting company. Jeff sustained his brain injury in Colorado where he was treated and continuously participates in rehabilitation.

Twice per week Jeff engages in a day program to be with other TBI survivors and those affected by multiple sclerosis where he takes classes such as cooking and art. He also works with several Independent Living Skills Trainers in-home and in the community to gain independence. Jeff likes to take long walks in the sunny Colorado weather, fish, and garden. He lives with his wife Cherie as well as his shitzu-poodle mix and two cats.

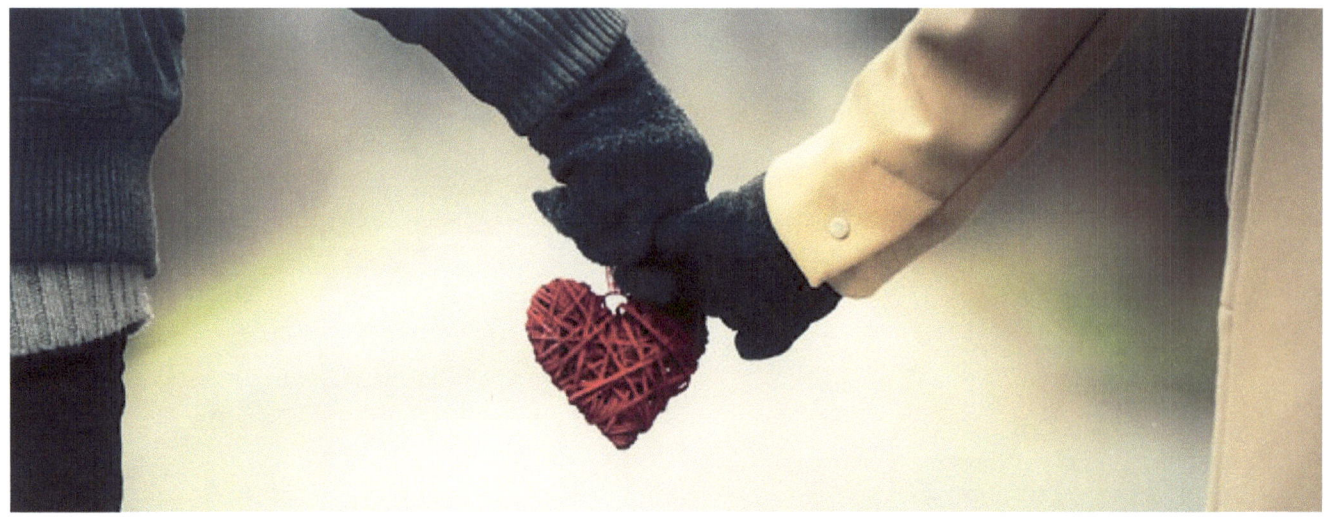

Transformed by Brain Injury

By Abby Maslin

On the morning before my 29-year-old husband went missing, he laced up his sneakers and went for a long run around the Tidal Basin, a few miles from our home in Washington, D.C. When he returned, I watched as he stood glistening with sweat and catching his breath in front of the bathroom mirror.

It's an image forever burned into my brain: my husband, TC, healthy. Full of energy. Radiating with life. I was as in love with him that morning as I was the night we met, back when I was a 22-year-old who believed good men were an urban myth and that there was surely no one in this world who could love me as big and fiercely as I was ready to love in return.

> "We promised to grow with each other, to stick together in sickness and in health, in failure and in triumph."

I was wrong. TC was every bit of the man I'd dreamed of meeting – handsome, ambitious, curious, and extraordinarily kind. Four years later we stood under a pear tree and took our vows as husband and wife. We promised to grow with each other, to stick together in sickness and in health, in failure and in triumph. A year after that we became parents to our son Jack, and it seemed impossible that the words "sickness" and "failure" could ever apply to our blessed family.

And then, three days after our third wedding anniversary, I awoke to a nightmare. TC was gone. My husband, an unfailingly responsible man (the kind of guy who rarely went out or drank too much), went to a baseball game with friends and never returned home. And for the first time in my life, I found myself praying for his irresponsibility. *Please let him be drunk on someone's couch. Please let him be passed out next to another woman.* These were the most promising scenarios I could think of. Anything else was inconceivably, irreversibly awful.

I told myself the words any ordinary person reassures themselves of when life's playbook takes an unexpected and potentially shocking direction: *this cannot be happening.* But it was. Seven blocks from my front stoop, where I stood with a police officer filing a missing person report, my husband, Jack's father, was being resuscitated after eight harrowing hours on the street. What had happened to TC was worse than anything I'd imagined: he'd been robbed, beaten on the head with a baseball bat and left to die.

Without permission, without notice, the first act of our marriage ended and the curtain rose on a new act, one that would revolve around three life altering words – *traumatic brain injury.* For 84 days, I sat by TC's hospital bedside as he recovered from a series of major surgeries. Among them, a craniectomy in which part of his skull was removed to depressurize his bleeding brain, a tracheostomy to get him through a near fatal case of pneumonia, and optic surgery to try and save the vision in his right eye.

I was swallowed up so entirely by each moment-to-moment crisis that I hardly had the capability to imagine the life waiting for us down the pipeline. And yet I was being warned at every turn. "If your husband survives," one doctor grimly conveyed, "you need to prepare yourself. He will not be the same person you remember."

As TC slowly woke from the fog of coma, the doctor's words rang true: this was not the man I married. There were the obvious and

> **"For 84 days, I sat by TC's hospital bedside as he recovered from a series of major surgeries."**

catastrophic changes; the cross-wiring of the brain had weakened his entire right side, leaving him with little mobility in his right extremities. Likewise, his right vision was seriously impaired, nearly gone. The most devastating impact of his injury, however, was in the part of the brain that controls language. TC could no longer speak or even understand the words that were being spoken to him. It is a condition known as *aphasia*, the inability to express or receive language.

There were also subtle changes. It was like TC had been transformed down to his very cellular make up. He no longer smelled the way I remembered: gone was the musky, wooded scent that reminded me of the fresh mountain air he had been born into nearly three decades earlier in rural West Virginia. Gone were the days of nuzzling myself in the crook of his arm just to soak up that comforting, delicious smell.

My new husband was a stranger – and a mute one at that – marked by the lingering odor of hospital disinfectant and an unruly beard that had been allowed to grow unbridled during the long months of his hospitalization.

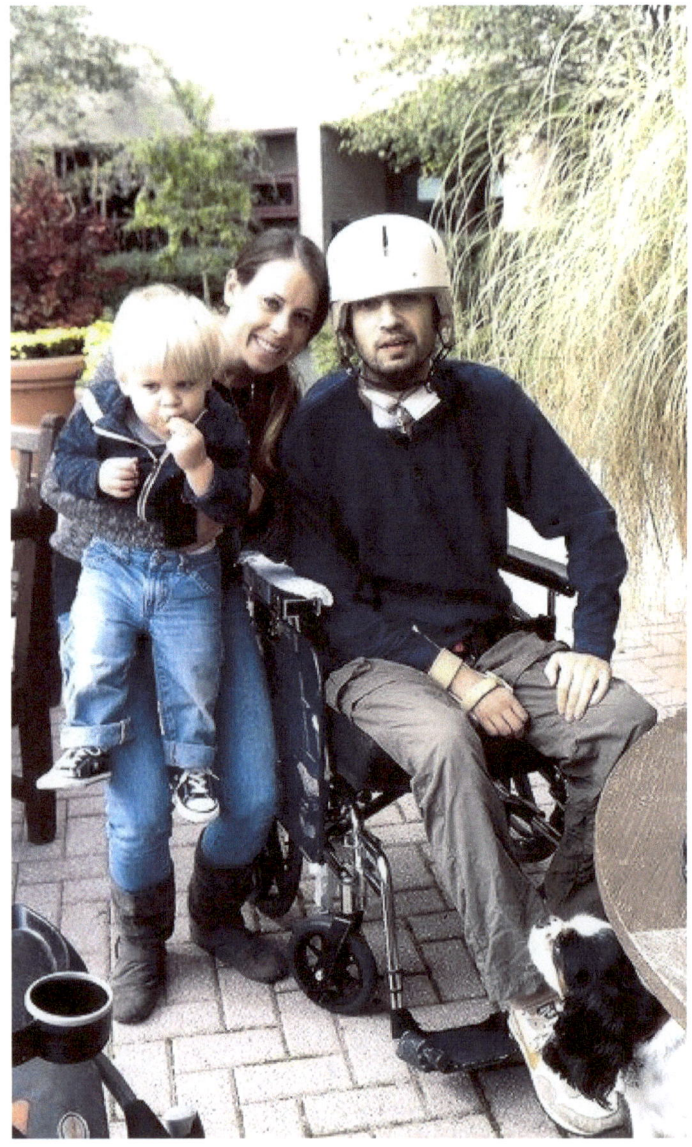

"I'm so sorry your life got ruined," remarked an acquaintance sympathetically, concern radiating from her wrinkled eyes.

"Thank you," I remember mumbling in response, unsure what to make of this brutally worded sentiment and the possible truth in it. Had my life been ruined? Was TC's brain injury the nail on the coffin of all our lives? And if so, what did this mean for our young son, to be the child of a disabled parent? What did it mean for the decades of marriage that lay ahead? Was I simply to sit in my misery for all that time – to accept the fate of a potentially joyless life?

I thought for a moment. *NO,* came the eventual answer from my hot-tempered soul. And again, *NO.* There was *no one*, no criminal, no doctor, no stranger – no injury that would determine if my life was ruined. That decision was in my hands alone. *I* would be the one to decide the outcome of my life.

Looking back, I don't think this woman will ever know how much I both hated and needed those words. For that day she ignited something in me that I will always consider a great gift: my will to fight. If there was any way to make lemonade from this horrifically tragic collection of lemons, anyway to save my little family and rebuild my marriage as I rebuilt my husband, I was determined to find it. I would accept it as the challenge of my lifetime.

Three months later, I took my new husband home from the hospital and the depth of my commitment was tested. TC was, as promised, unable to walk without a wheelchair or cane, unable to communicate anything more sophisticated than a few simple sentences, and severely limited in the use of his right arm.

We quickly fell into the role of silent roommates. Without language to connect our experiences, there was little glue left in the relationship. Interactions as simple as making a grocery list together were painful, confusing, and drawn out, making it nearly impossible to discuss anything as complex as the circumstances of TC's assault or the loneliness that had pervaded our family dynamic.

For months, as TC participated in intense therapies to help him regain his speech and motor skills, I fell into a deep depression. I laid in bed at night talking to my best friend, my husband, as if he were dead and in heaven instead of passed out in slumber right beside me. I lingered in each phase of ambiguous grief, unsure how to explain my loneliness and the choking sense of loss I felt each day, even though my husband was still alive.

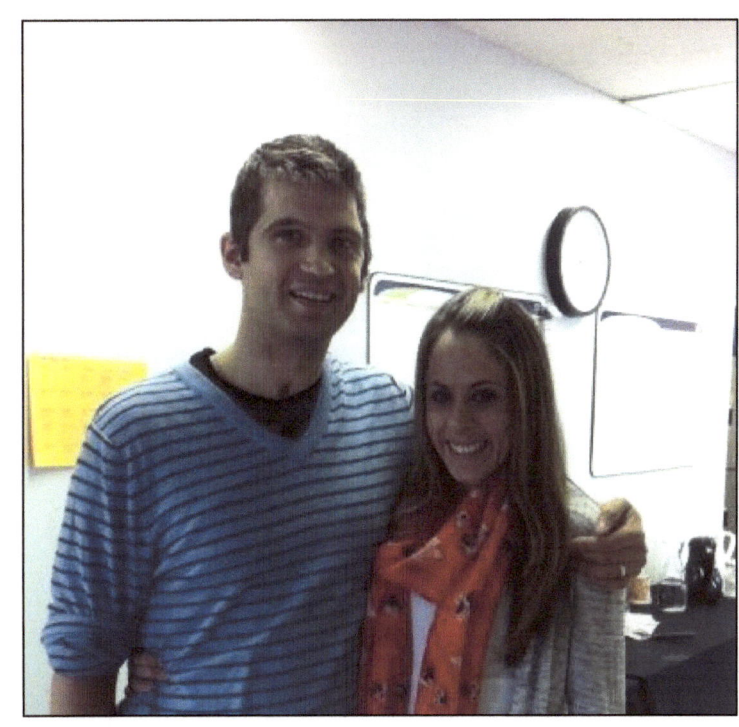

I missed him. With every fiber of my being, I tried to cling to happy memories of the life we once shared. And even though it hadn't been a perfect life, full of its own minor struggles, I could no longer remember any of the challenges. My life before had been pure, and I innocent, a stranger to the black hole of grief and heartbreak so many of us stumble through during our lifetimes.

I looked at my new husband, fiercely determined to get well, even though simple tasks like setting the table or changing our son's diaper fatigued him for hours, and I began to ask myself the hard questions about love – questions I had blown my way past as a 27-year-old skipping down the aisle.

Why do we love the people we love? Is it because of how they look? How they make us feel? The things they can do or the security they bring us? Or is it their intellect, their humor, the stuff we don't have words for – a quality or set of qualities that transcend language?

I had promised to make lemonade out of lemons, but along the way I had fallen victim to self-pity. I was so entrenched in my grief over everything I'd lost that I was ignoring what was right in front of me: a man so determined to get his life back I'd catch him doing leg lifts at the sink as he washed the dishes after dinner. A man who may not have had the words to say *I love you*, but showed it in every small and important way that counted.

Yes, he had been changed, but not by his own volition. And so I decided: the most loving, dedicated thing I could do to honor the great man TC once was and the great man he was striving to be in this new life was to change too. My new husband deserved a new wife.

Brain injury demands we abandon our former expectations and learn to look at life through an innovative lens. The more I thought about it, the more I realized my love for TC was not rooted in the way he looked, his successful career, or even his natural athleticism.

I did not love him for the way he played guitar or the beautifully crafted love letters he wrote. I loved him for something that transcended all that – something that existed beyond his abilities and even his words. I loved him for his spirit. His determination to live. The spark of compassion and gentle humility that exists at the very core of his being. And brain injury had not broken that. It had only stripped everything else away, allowing me to meet my real husband for the very first time.

Six years have passed since TC's assault and our "new normal" looks deceptively similar to the life we had before. We have a lovely home, two healthy children, and more blessings than I ever could have dared to hope for in those early days of brain injury. But an image alone does not tell the complete story.

It has taken extraordinary perseverance and a lot of help from others to rebuild our lives from the ground up. Through the frustration, the disappointment, and the setbacks, TC has fought relentlessly, filling me with endless pride and admiration. These days he is walking, speaking

Six years have passed since TC's assault and our "new normal" looks deceptively similar to the life we had before.

with clarity, and back at work. Our marriage has survived some dark, brutal days, but we are committed to one another, bound by a respect and appreciation for each other's strength. It may not sound sexy or romantic, but if I've learned anything about marriage, it's this: real love demands the best of us. If we're willing to get in the trenches and roll up our sleeves, we may be surprised by the depth of love we experience in return.

This life will always be a fight. After all, disability does not just go away. TC's injury has shaped our lives and transformed the dynamic of each and every interaction we have, leaving open the possibility of a very uncertain future. But it does not own us. And it certainly hasn't ruined our lives. Instead, brain injury has been a teacher – guiding us into a life centered around the things that truly matter, growing our gratitude in every way, and reminding us to never take a moment of our time together for granted.

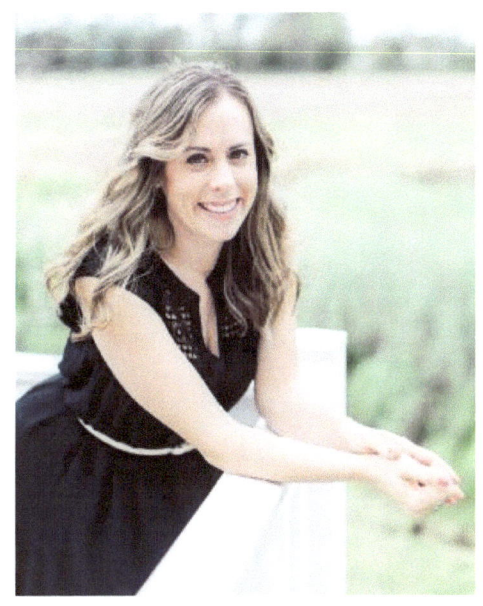

Meet Abby Maslin

Abby Maslin is a writer and a public school teacher. She holds master's degrees in education and creative arts therapy. After her husband suffered a severe TBI as a result of a brutal assault in their Washington, DC neighborhood, Abby began documenting their family's struggle on her personal blog.

She currently serves as a regular contributor to the website Brainline.org and is the author of the recently released bestselling memoir, Love You Hard. You can learn more about Abby on her website: abbymaslin.com.

Join our Facebook Family

What do almost 30,000 people from 60 countries and five continents all have in common? They are all members of our vibrant Facebook family at ⓕ/TBIHopeandInspiration

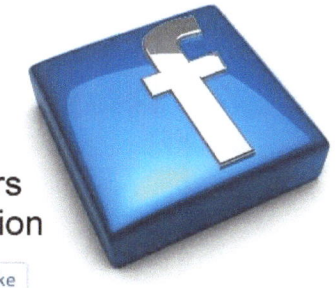

A Help Button Should Go Where You Go!

"Hello, this is MobileHelp. How may I assist you?"

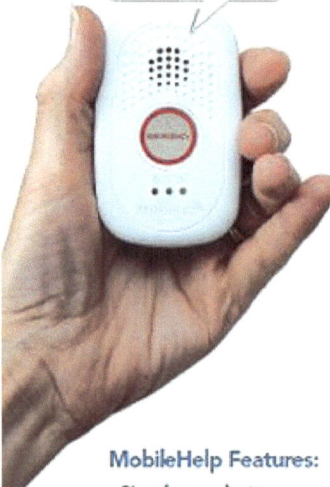

To be truly independent your personal emergency device needs to work on the go.

MobileHelp® allows you to summon emergency help 24 hours a day, 365 days a year by simply pressing your personal help button. Unlike traditional systems that only work inside your home, MobileHelp's medical alert system extends help beyond the home. Now you can participate in all your favorite activities such as gardening, taking walks, shopping and traveling all with the peace of mind of having a personal medical alert system with you. MobileHelp, the "on-the-go" help button, is powered by one of the nation's largest cellular networks, so there's virtually no limit to your help button's range.* With our GPS feature activated, we can send help to you, even when you can't talk or tell us where you are.

No landline? No Problem! While traditional medical alert systems require a landline, with MobileHelp's system, a landline is not necessary. Whether you are home or away from home, a simple press of your help button activates your system, providing the central station with your information and location. Our trained emergency operators will know who you are and where you are located.

If you're one of the millions of people that have waited for a medical alert service because it didn't fit your lifestyle, or settled for a traditional system even though it only worked in the home, then we welcome you to try MobileHelp. Experience peace of mind in the home or on the go.

MobileHelp Features:

- Simple one-button operation
- Affordable service
- Amplified 2-way voice communication
- 24/7/365 access to U.S. based operators
- GPS location detection
- Available Nationwide

As seen on:

  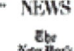

Unlike 'stay-at-home' emergency systems MobileHelp protects you:		
Places where your Help Button will work	MobileHelp	Traditional Help Buttons
Home	✓	✓
On a Walk	✓	✗
On Vacation	✓	✗
At the Park	✓	✗
Shopping	✓	✗

Order Now & Receive a FREE Lockbox!

Place your door key in this box so that emergency personnel can get help to you even faster.

$29.95 Value

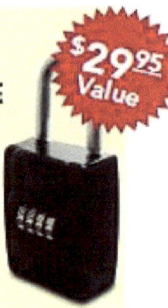

Optional Fall Button™

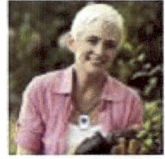

The automatic fall detect pendant that works **WHERE YOU GO!**

MobileHelp

1-800-371-2132

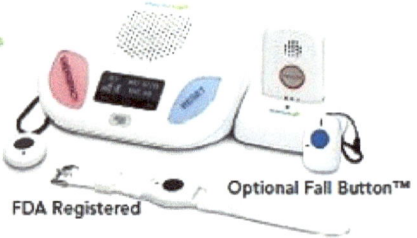

FDA Registered

Optional Fall Button™

See What I See

By Tracie Massie

You ask me how I make it day to day
I struggle to put into words what I want to say
I know you're concerned about what seems to be my destiny
But when you look in his eyes you can't see what I see
The baby I carried, what a beautiful sight
To see him asleep on his dad's chest at night
The boy that did the "hard jobs" for his Pop and worked steady
For the man who was gone before we were ready
The teenager that took pride in his high school football team
With a big future ahead, or so it would seem
Then came the call when I heard his coach say
"There's been an accident, come right away"
I raced to the hospital feeling panic and fear
Wondering what I would find when I arrived there
The doctors were great, the nurses so good
They tried to prepare me for this new phase of parenthood
There were so many things left unsaid
But there's nothing to prepare you for an injury involving the head
They never told me the boy that I raised was gone
It's a very different person that I call "son"
Anxiety, hot temper, health problems galore
Yet he's alive, I have that to be thankful for
Yes I get tired and discouraged too
Without my husband and family I don't know what I would do
Remember he tries though at times not hard enough
Other's lives help me see mine could be so much more rough
So next time you ask me how I put up with what I do
I hope you will see the boy I see too

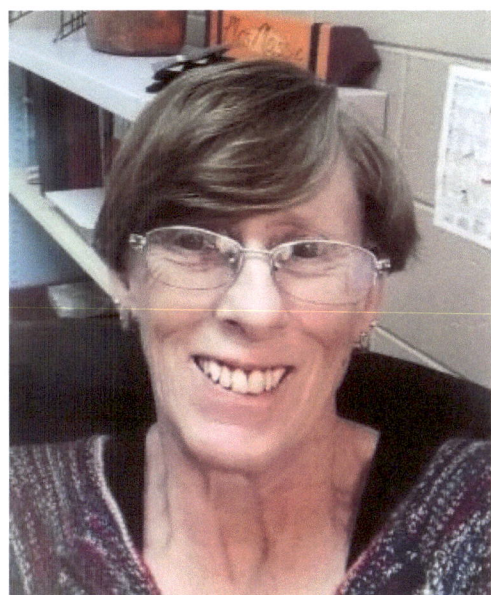

Meet Tracie

"My name is Tracie Massie, I live in Darbyville, Ohio and work for our local school as teacher's aide for special needs and IEP students. I am the mother of a TBI survivor. My son's TBI occurred when he pulled out in front of a semi in 2006. He was in a coma for three weeks at Grant Medical Center and spent six weeks in rehab at Nationwide Children's Hospital. He has suffered two more TBI's since, one due to another car accident and the third happened when he was jumped by three people and kicked in the head repeatedly.

I worked in the healthcare field almost my entire adult life, which was a huge help when it came to caring for my son after the accident but I really believe his TBI prepared me for the job I have now working with special needs students. I have found that it has awakened a passion inside me for helping do all I can for them and be an advocate for them when needed. I wrote this poem in response to friends and family members asking me how I make it through each day."

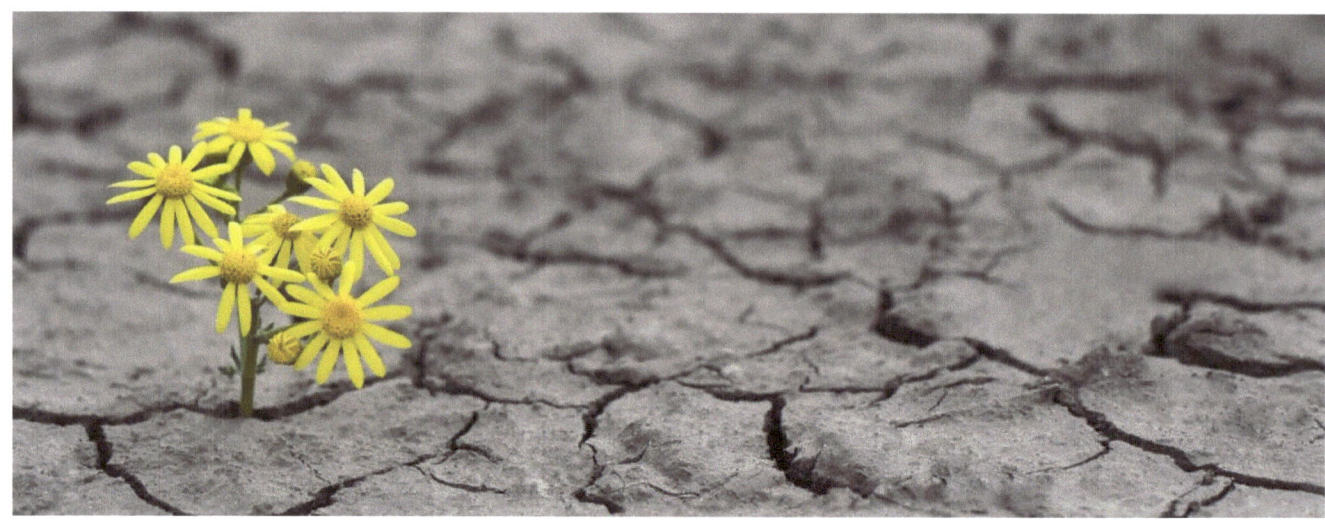

The Fierce Heart of Hope

By Nicole Bingaman

We gathered in the dimly lit corridor of Geisinger Medical Center as Taylor entered the first hours following his initial craniectomy. The waiting room closest to the AICU was closed, so we created a makeshift area in the hallway. Waiting areas were available on other floors, but we needed to be close by.

Around the third day of Taylor's hospitalization, a pastor came to visit. Stepping off the elevator and into our makeshift space, he spoke, "I understand things look pretty hopeless here." Emotions were running high and his words fell on our ears in a way that caused us to be defensive.

> "I did not have the energy to entertain the words of a stranger. I was pouring all I had into my prayers for Taylor."

We were allowed to acknowledge how bleak things were. However, we did not welcome a mere acquaintance giving voice to our despair. We knew Taylor may not survive and things were leaning in that direction, but to hear the word "hopeless" in regard to our situation was too much.

After the pastor's statement, I shut him out. My father tells me he went on to share thoughts that were more compassionate. However, his opening words halted the idea of my hearing any more. I was emotionally fatigued and raw. I did not have the energy to entertain the words of a stranger. I was pouring all I had into my prayers for Taylor.

Upon reflection, I know this man's words were not intended to deliver the blow they did. But something else arose from his utterance of disparity. After he left, we used our anger at his words to rally our own hope.

Around the same time, Avery (our middle son) brought one of my sweatshirts into Taylor's room. He whispered, "Let's leave this by Tayl." On the front of the sweatshirt was one word… **HOPE**, and on the back, two words… **changes everything.** Avery wanted to place the shirt across Taylor's body, but we had to settle for the chair situated closest to him. Taylor was incredibly fragile and our interactions with him were limited.

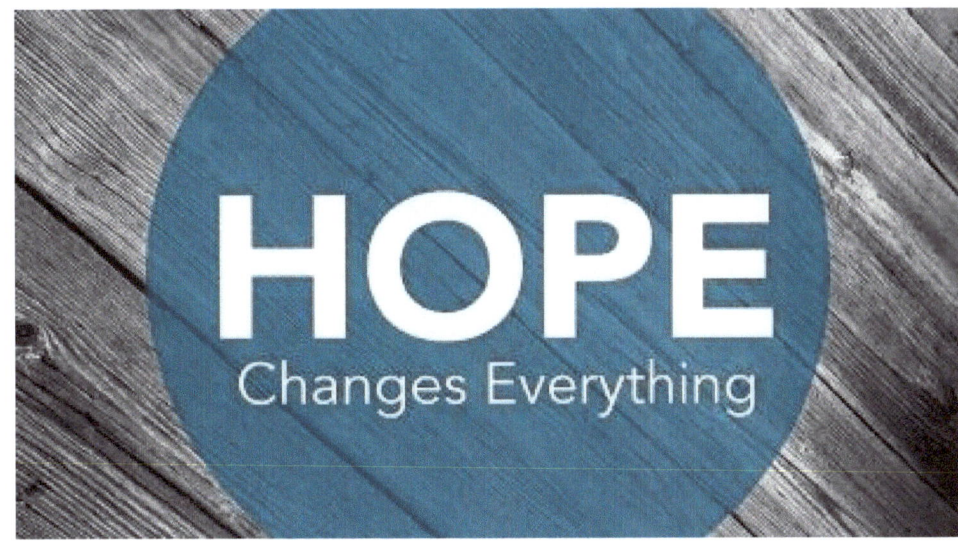

The shirt was something I created years before in response to losing my stepbrother, Ralph. Ralph was shot in the head during a random drive-by shooting. He died immediately as a result of the spinning bullet that entered his brain. His death became a doorway to something in my own soul. The idea of hope being stronger than death sat with me and I explored it. This exploration was born out of witnessing my stepmother's grief and the desire for some sense of light to come out of the darkness of Ralph's murder.

Nine years later, as my son fought for his life, I knew I was given a gift that was robbed from my stepmom… a chance to say goodbye… precious moments with my son. Even if they were the last, I needed to be grateful for each one of them.

I knew hope could exist in the chasm of despair. The shirt was a tangible reminder. Hope sat close to Taylor on a garment I had created. Admittedly, hope was far more difficult to cling to now that it was my son fighting for his life.

Hope is complicated. It represents believing something can improve, despite the current state of circumstances. It also means having the courage to believe when things appear hopeless. I have become well acquainted with the infinite value of hope, but also the tightrope on which it teeters.

Seven months later, our family gathered around the dinner table. Taylor had survived weeks in the ICU, lived at a rehab for several months and was participating in outpatient therapies at home. He had relearned to walk, speak, get dressed and more. We were sitting with someone who embodied perseverance and determination and yet we were depleted of hope.

To say things felt horrible would be a tremendous understatement. Each one of us felt an immeasurable sadness, frustration, and anger about what was now unfolding. Taylor was unexpectedly regressing. Earlier that day, we learned that Taylor's body was rejecting the piece of his skull that had previously been replaced. We were going to face another series of unknowns. After surviving more than we ever imagined, the possibility was again presented that we could lose all we had fought so hard for.

We could lose even more of Taylor… and ourselves. Taylor tired quickly and did not last long at the dinner table. We returned him to his bedroom and reconvened at the table. If hope were a picture hanging on the wall of our home, it would have appeared visibly smashed, dismantled, and barely hanging on. We were too exhausted to hold onto hope. The situation screamed at us, like a drill sergeant trying to break a cadet, "Let hope go!"

I recall the heaviness in the room. The fear was palpable. We were all full of anguish. Months of emotional turmoil topped by exhaustion, and now the idea we might have to do it again. It appeared that defeat was replacing our reservoir of hope.

My youngest son spoke. Tanner was a high school senior. He was an athlete who, despite his small stature and lighter weight, was a respected running back, known for fighting through a tough line. Tanner knew how to fight something that appeared larger and stronger than you. He shared this idea, "If we lose hope, we lose everything. Without hope, we might as well give up." He was challenging us. This was a plainly spoken reminder to us. Hope was too valuable to lose.

We didn't discuss how we were going to get this thing called hope back. And as life with brain injury would have it, hope would come and go and would be tested tirelessly through countless ordeals. But in time, I have learned to let the whisper of hope be louder than the shout of despair. I can tell you it takes a lot of practice and patience and sometimes I still miss the mark.

But I still conclude that hope changes everything, most of all the heart in which it resides.

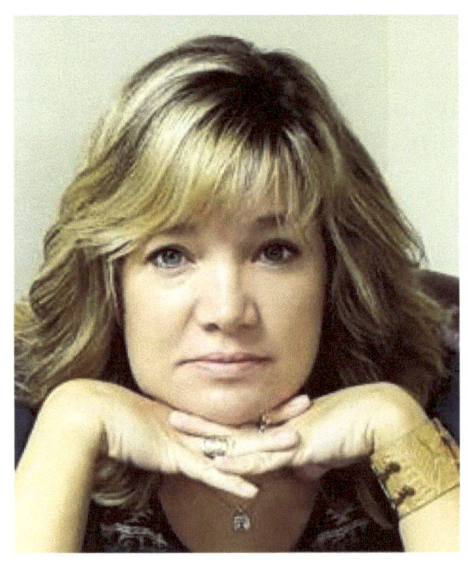

Meet Nicole Bingaman

"Along with being a caregiver, I am a caseworker for the Commonwealth of Pennsylvania. Prior to that I taught art, English and Life Skills to at-risk youth in an alternative education setting. I believe that all people deserve compassion and understanding. Within that belief is where I've found my most important role as a caregiver and mother. I live with my husband, Keith, and our sons, Taylor, our strong survivor, Tanner, a banjo playing philosophy major, and Avery, who recently accepted a position with the Peace Corps in Africa, and my adored dog, Ginger."

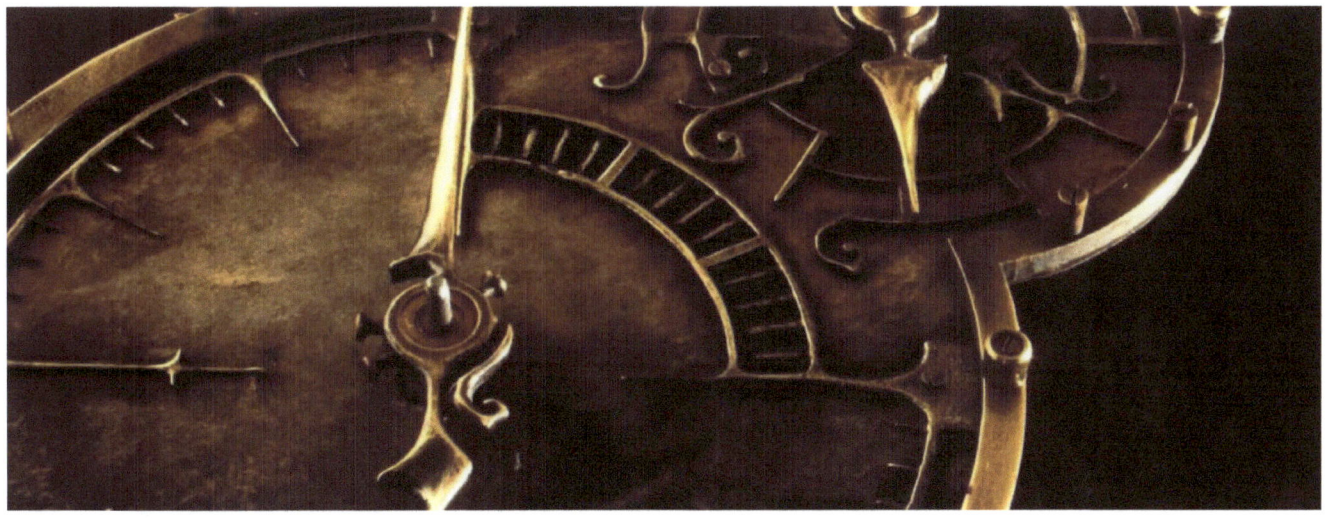

The Double-Edged Sword of Time

By David A. Grant

With very little fanfare, and with a large serving of cake late last year, I crossed the threshold into my ninth year as a brain injury survivor. As the years continue to pass, new perspectives come that are only possible with the passage of time.

During the first year or two after my brain injury, there was a mass exodus of friends and family from my life. It was unexpected. It was shocking. However, time now reveals that it is quite typical. In *The TBI Guide* by Dr. Glen Johnson, he shares that most brain injury survivors lose up to 90% of their closer friends within the first year after an injury. The reasons are not as complicated as you might think. Like many others, my personality changed rather dramatically after my brain injury. Simply put, I became a different person. Human nature being what it is, people shun the unfamiliar.

> "Like many others, my personality changed rather dramatically after my brain injury."

They shunned me.

But Dr. Johnson goes on to share that the void left when people depart is eventually filled with new friends, those who only know the post-injury person. So it has been for me. I find myself today with some of the strongest relationships I've had in my life. Many are with other members of the survivor community, but many are with people outside the realm of brain injury. To them, I am the only David they know. They never knew the earlier version of me.

Those friends who stuck by me through all of this have come to accept me as I am today – quirky, forgetful, and different than the David they originally befriended. Though no one says it directly, enough time has passed so that these cherished souls have forgotten a lot about who I used to be. To them, I'm just David.

While at first glance this all sounds good, there is a double-edged sword to all this. Over 90% of the time, external symptoms of my brain injury are non-existent. I can conduct myself reasonably well in public and my verbal and emotional filters function better than they have in years. To those who know nothing of my back-story, I look and act somewhat normal.

Brain injury is not called an *invisible disability* by chance. Even on my best days, I still have very significant challenges. Trying to follow conversations, especially when there are a few people involved, is very tough. I find myself playing the role of constant listener, lest I speak and reveal my disability.

At the times when I do jump into conversations, I do so with great care and restraint. I speak slowly and methodically, thinking about every word before I speak it. This is a fallback to a technique that I developed in 2011, when I abruptly lost the ability to speak clearly.

Think the word. Say the word. Think the word. Say the word.

Like an athlete whose skills are fine-tuned over time, I practice this technique to this day, but at a speed quickly enough so that most never notice. But I notice.

Herein lies the challenge of being a long-term survivor. People close to me often think I am "over" all my brain injury challenges. Those new in my life did not see my struggles during my first couple of years.

> **"Trying to follow conversations, especially when there are a few people involved, is very tough."**

Those who have known me for a long time mistakenly think that I am okay now. It's understandable perceptions like this that make ME put almost inhuman expectations on myself. The internal monologue often says things like, "You have been doing this long enough to be beyond having big challenges."

Moreover, when those challenges happen, I feel devastated thinking that I should do better. I fail to cut myself slack and look not at how far I have come, but rather, I focus on the deficiencies still at hand.

Complicated? You tell me.

So much of my day-to-day life as a brain injury survivor requires more effort than most anyone will ever know. I work harder and accomplish less. I try to stay focused but distract easily. I try to live as I once did and experience the futility of it. I walk through crowds of the uninjured and feel apart from much of humanity, different than, and less than those without a brain injury. Most of the time, none of this can be seen by anyone.

The more "normal" I appear, the greater the gap between what you see and what I know my truth to be.

I try to always end on a positive, uplifting note. Today I have to dig a bit deeper for this. If my soul-level sharing today helps one person to feel less isolated and less alone in their own struggles, then a greater good has been realized. If a family member or caregiver can better understand a loved one, that same greater good has been realized.

To all who now live lives affected by brain injury, I can share that life does indeed get easier over time, but at times like this…well, it's complicated.

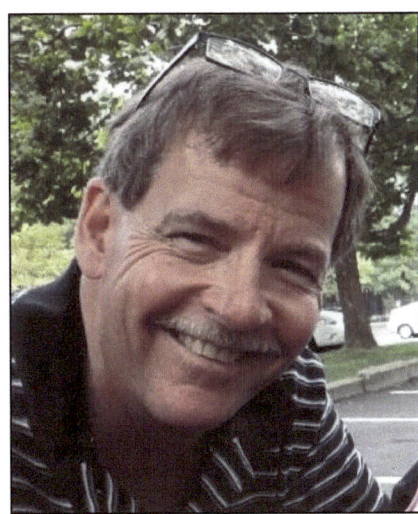

Meet David A. Grant

David A. Grant is a freelance writer based out of southern New Hampshire and the publisher of HOPE Magazine. He is the author of Metamorphosis, Surviving Brain Injury.

He is also a contributing author to Chicken Soup for the Soul, Recovering from Traumatic Brain Injuries. David is a BIANH Board Member. David is a regular contributing writer to Brainline.org, a PBS sponsored website.

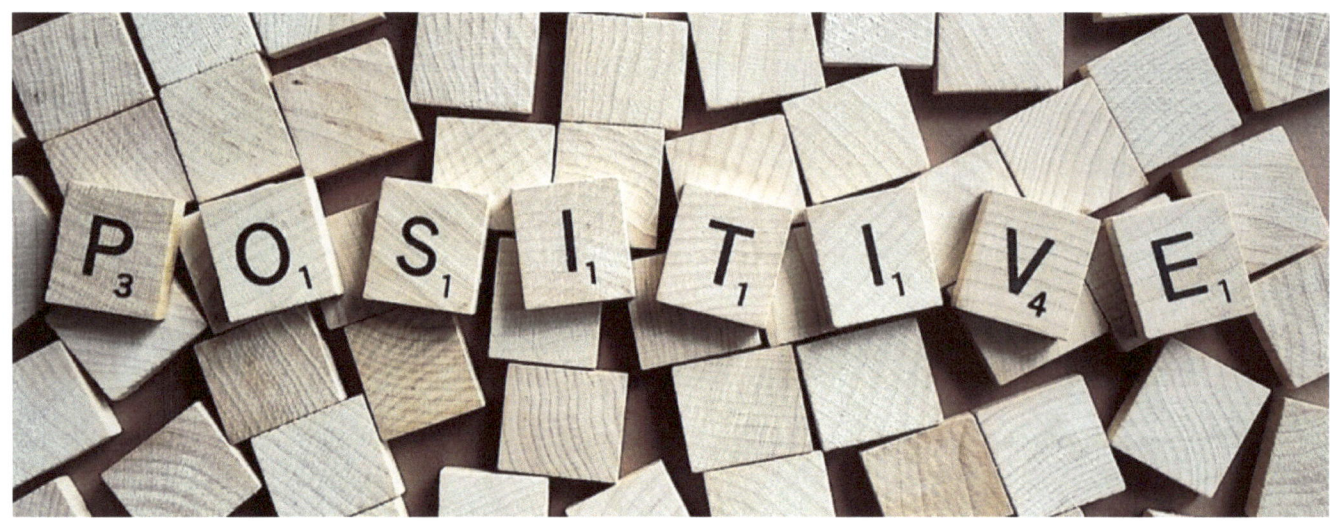

Positive Things

By Tobie-Lynn Andrade

Life changes after brain injury. I have learned many positive ways to view things that happen after a TBI. I have found a humorous and humble approach to being happier that I would like to share.

You will learn who is real in your life.
Honestly, the false and good weather friends will drift away and family and friends who remain during your worst days will celebrate your best. You will be stronger and won't be carrying the weight of acquaintances and people who don't really want to be there.

You will forget things.
Little things, big things, in-between things. You will forget what you are doing while you are doing it. You will forget to finish sentences, eat meals, and endings to books and movies. Take it in stride. You will spend less money on books and movies, because you can reread and watch the ones you have and have the experience of doing it for the first time, a lot! You will also find the bad memories dim, hospital stays, friends that have slipped away, those weeks of depression – they will slowly fade and become less of a stress.

> "You will spend less money on books and movies, because you can reread and watch the ones you have."

Vision issues.

You probably didn't realize you would have issues. I didn't expect it. Whether it be floaters in your vision, lack of depth perception or sensitivity to light, own it! Think of how boring that plain beige wall is at the doctor's office, now look how speckled and interesting it looks with all those squiggly lines. Rock those sunglasses or bifocals, unleash your inner Elton John and be fabulous in your specs.

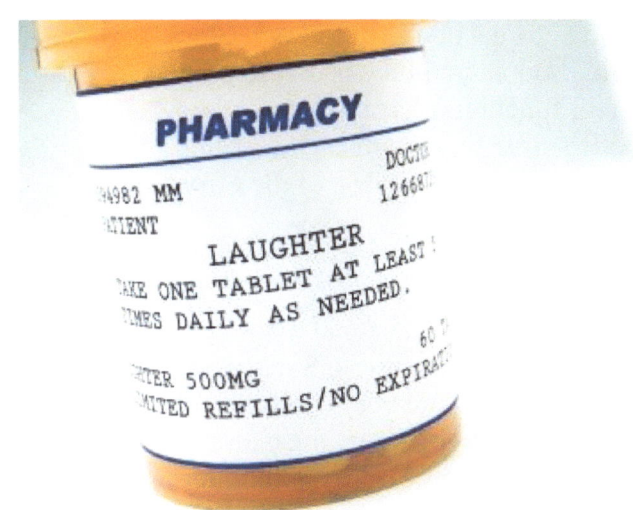

Not working.

Sure, the financial aspect of not working or collecting disability sucks, but no more terrible bosses, long meetings, awful coworkers. Also, you are now on your own schedule. Don't shy away when people ask what you do for work, tell them you get to stay in your pj's all day on a weekday, or have a nap when others are working through lunch. Remember every part of working you dreaded and know it's no longer an issue. Take up hobbies during the time you set aside to focus on your career, read those novels you always wanted to, binge on whole television series, use the time you used to spend at work on yourself.

You are now an expert.

Yep. People spend thousands of dollars and years and energy to try and understand what you are going through, and you are living it. No one knows your brain, your body, your experience better than you. You remind doctors what you are seeing them for, you pass on information to agencies and insurance companies so they can do their job. Your answers are in demand. Not only that, but you will learn more about medical forms, and special mailing instructions and appeal allowances than you ever thought possible. Add initials after your name, make up a title like mine: Tobie-Lynn Andrade "B.I.E." Or, if you are too shy to add Brain Injury Expert after your name, use a humbler title like "Self-Awareness Award Winner, six years running."

You learn to value the little things.

Health is something I didn't consciously take for granted, but every migraine, seizure, or neurological issue that has come since my TBI makes me ever so grateful for the good moments when my body doesn't seem to be betraying me. I also find pleasure in getting snail mail and celebrate many small moments like reading a chapter aloud without stuttering. Embrace the happiness, smell the flowers, take time for joy. You have survived every bad day until today.

Physical trials don't define us.

Some of us are walking, some are sitting, and some are bed-ridden. Whatever abilities remain, however varied, are ours. Use what tools you can to live life fully. Make jokes at your own expense. Watch Forrest Gump teach the King how to shake that pelvis and own your moves. There is more than one awkward dancer made famous on YouTube. If you drift to the right when walking down a hallway, start on the left side so you don't brush the wall. Know your limits and needs and use your environment to succeed. There are countless tools and tips and therapies to help you along. Use whatever works, forget about that foot dragging or your eyelid drooping and focus on the parts of you that still function. I have a friend who types with one single finger and each word he types is more meaningful because of the effort he puts into it.

Depending on others.
Be it driving, shopping, or personal hygiene tasks, we need help in some areas. Sure, it isn't ideal, especially if you were very independent before your injury. But you know the people who are still here want to be, so lean on them for support. Enjoy being chauffeured, having meals delivered and getting your hair done. Remember it makes people feel good to help you. Don't be embarrassed when others help count change or guide you; be thankful you don't have to struggle alone. Release your inner princess and ring the bell for your tea, and don't feel guilty about it.

People's expectations are lower now.
And that is OK. You might exceed them or miss them altogether on your journey, but those who love and support you don't expect you to function like you did Before. That is a good thing. You will realize the pressure you feel to perform at a certain level is your own, others are happy to ride at your speed. You can also make their expectations more realistic; if you are able to speak for yourself when meeting a new person tell them they don't have to ask your caregivers. Inform others about what you are able to do and what you need help with. Many an awkward situation can be avoided by clear communication.

You will laugh at yourself.
It will happen when you least expect it, during your bleakest moments, you will fumble a word or replace it with something entirely wrong and hilarious and will laugh your butt off. Others will laugh with you if they see you laughing,

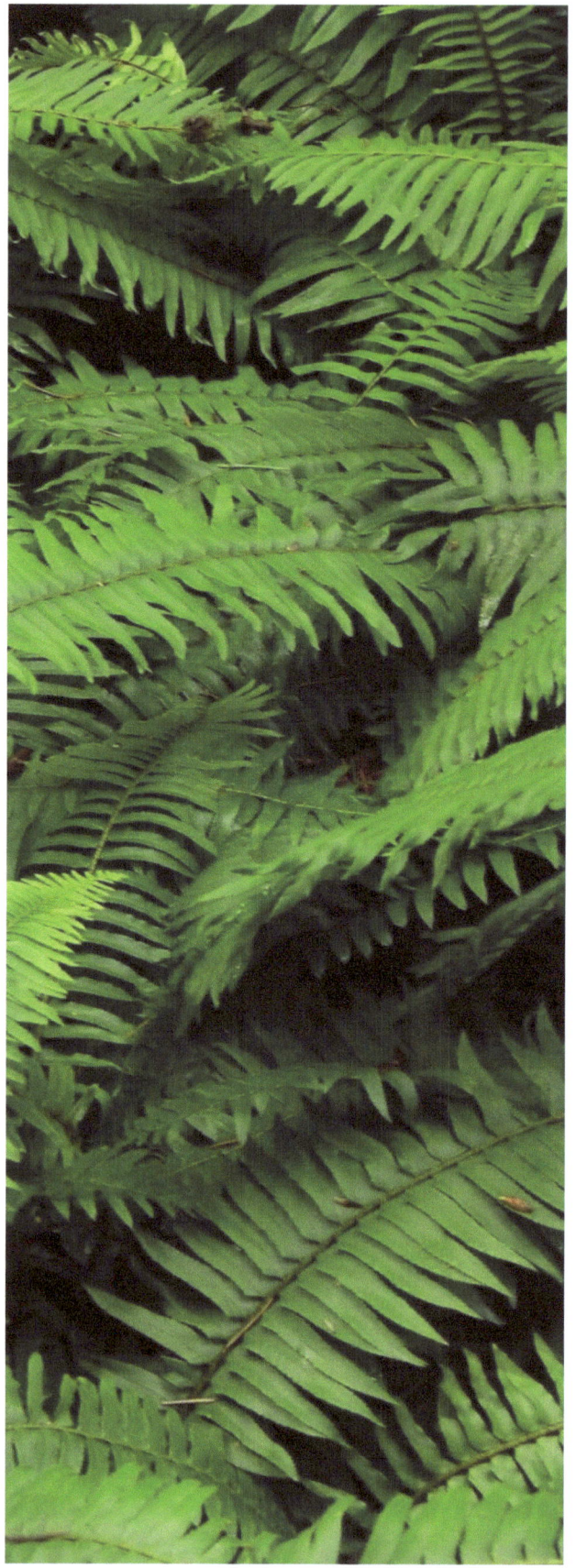

and you will have funny memories to recall (or to listen to others recall, because you know, the memory thing!) I have had some very amusing trips and slips and funky dance moves while learning to navigate and more than my share of awkward verbal slip ups. Shake it off, make a joke, smile, laughter really is the best medicine.

Bravery.
Unlike anything you ever went through before, you will find inner strength to draw on and you will be braver than you ever thought possible. Maybe not in your exact current situation, but you will overcome and succeed and realize you belong at the round table, or in Gryffindor House, or that you deserve to lead a country because You Are Brave. Why? Because you are here, reading this article, fighting this fight, and living. That also makes you pretty darned awesome.

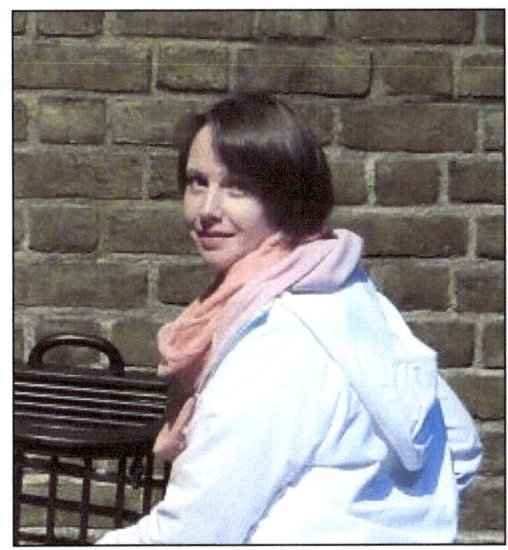

Meet Tobie-Lynn Andrade

Tobie-Lynn is a lifelong fan of reading and an avid crafter, as well as a huge Harry Potter geek. She is recovering from a grade three concussion with front left lobe damage and post-concussion syndrome with seizures.

Tobie-Lynn is using natural medicines and methods to heal from her injuries, and the Harry Potter stories to help herself heal. One of her greatest moments in life was going to England where the Harry Potter series was filmed and standing with her husband on the actual bridge used in the films.

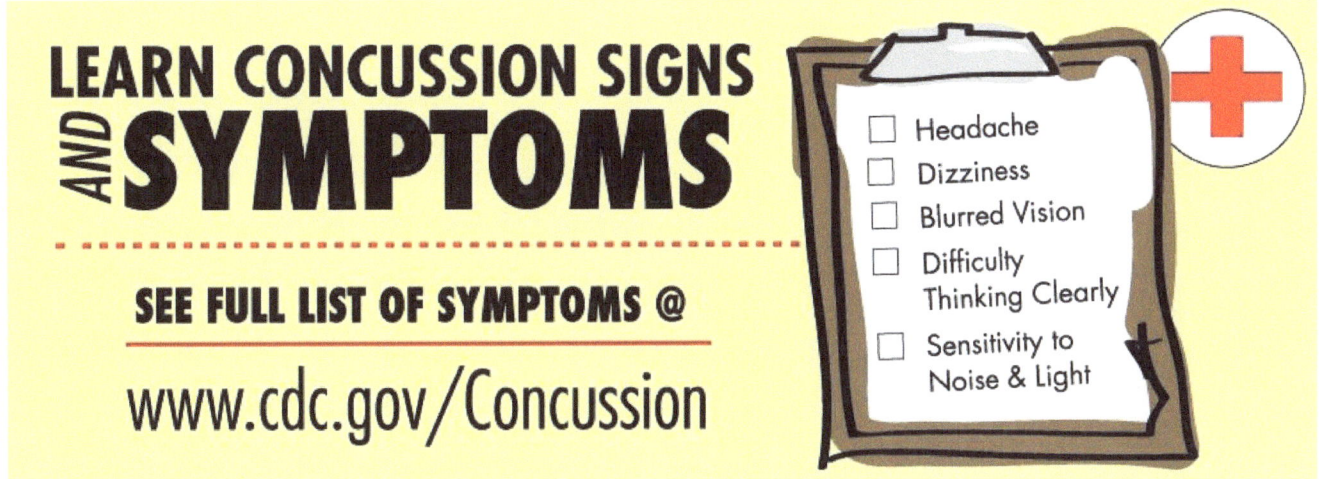

LEARN CONCUSSION SIGNS AND SYMPTOMS

SEE FULL LIST OF SYMPTOMS @

www.cdc.gov/Concussion

☐ Headache
☐ Dizziness
☐ Blurred Vision
☐ Difficulty Thinking Clearly
☐ Sensitivity to Noise & Light

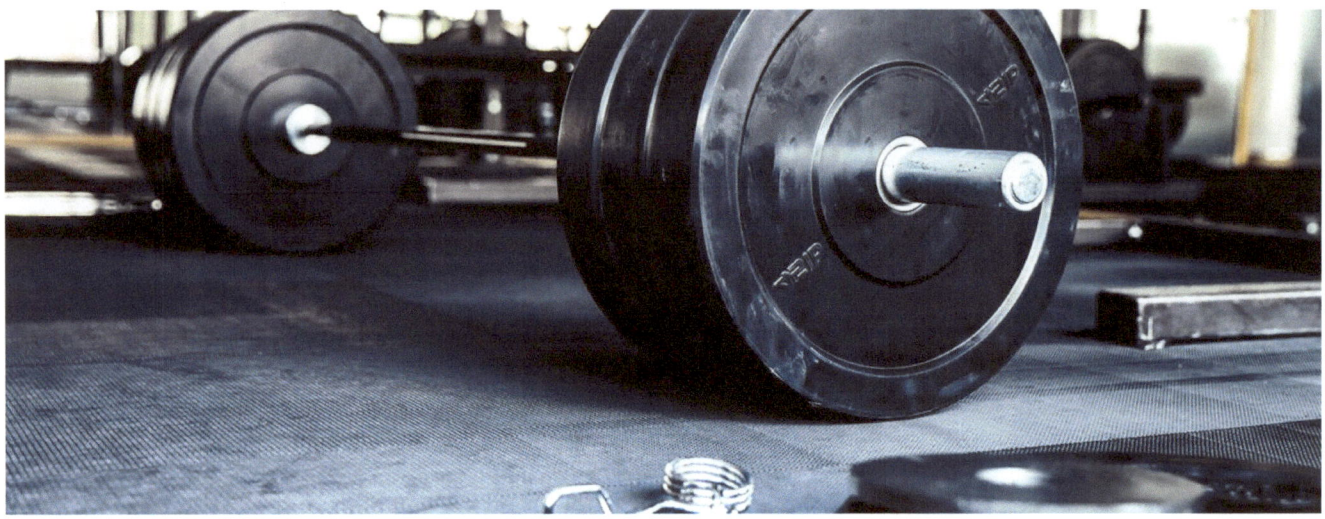

Two Years Stong

By Kiana Kay

After a long afternoon of shopping with two young children, Brent and his girlfriend Sarah decided it was time to head home. They strapped Arianna, 21 months old at the time and Aiden, 1 month old, into their car seats and began driving home. Only one town away from home, they came around a turn when a white utility van swerved over the double yellow lines and collided into their Ford Focus, crashing along the driver's side of the car as well as on top of it, forcing the car to flip onto its passenger side. Upon impact Brent was thrown from the driver's seat on to his girlfriend in the passenger seat.

His left elbow was shattered, his C Spine was injured, and he was knocked unconscious. In the backseat, Arianna was unconscious and bleeding. When the car flipped to its side, a window was shattered causing Arianna's head to be cut open. Both Brent and Arianna suffered severe brain injuries amongst other injuries. Sarah's arm was broken when Brent fell on her, but she was fine overall; baby Aiden was in the backseat miraculously unharmed.

> "Both Brent and Arianna suffered severe brain injuries amongst other injuries."

When ambulances arrived, Arianna was revived on-scene and then driven to the nearest airport where she was airlifted to Dartmouth Hitchcock Medical Center in New Hampshire, placed into a medically induced coma, and taken into emergency surgery for her open brain injury. Brent was driven to the nearest hospital where he was then airlifted to Dartmouth as well.

I couldn't imagine there being anything more alarming than the call you receive being told your child has been in a severe accident and is not breathing. Sitting on the basement stairs of her house, having a casual conversation with her husband, my mother received a call from Sarah but there was no noise. After saying Sarah's name three times, Sarah replied with a scream just before the phone got disconnected. A few minutes later Sarah called my mother back using Brent's phone, frantically explaining what happened, she told my mother that Brent and Arianna were not breathing and that they had been in an accident. I couldn't imagine the amount of fear, panic, disbelief, and helplessness that may have overcome my mother's body in that moment.

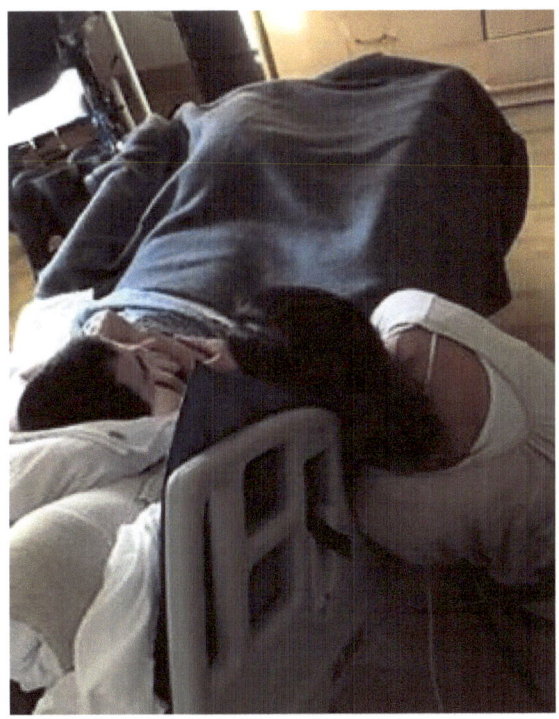

She got into her car and rushed toward where Brent was. Once she arrived, she watched as he was lifted up by the helicopter. Unsure what condition he was in, she headed to the hospital he was being flown to. Sarah was brought to the nearest hospital with Aiden to have her broken arm casted and for Aiden to be examined for injuries. The accident happened in Gilford, NH an hour and a half or so from Lebanon, NH where Dartmouth Hospital is located.

At the hospital, Arianna was in brain surgery for five hours and had a pressure bolt put into her head so that doctors and nurses could measure her intracranial pressure. Brent was brought into the E.R. Trauma bay where nurses were shuffling around placing ice packs on him to get the swelling to go down all over his body. Doctors were considering whether or not they should amputate his left arm because his elbow was shattered so badly, but they decided against it. He was placed on a ventilator due to collapsed lungs. Twelve hours later Brent was taken into surgery where surgeons inserted a drainage tube into his skull to drain spinal fluid as well as a pressure bolt to monitor the spike in intracranial pressure. He was covered with different tubes and wires and swollen from head to toe.

Following surgery, Brent was moved to the Intensive Care Unit because he was in critical condition. Once the chaos had calmed down, doctors came out into the waiting room to get my mother to allow her to finally see Brent. While standing beside Brent, my mother was informed that Brent had suffered a Diffused Axonal Injury, a brain injury that only 10% of people survive and that they were not sure if Brent would even survive it. The ICU staff and PICU staff were so incredibly caring and amazing when working with Brent and Arianna – they are the reason Brent and Arianna are alive today and our family will be forever grateful!

On January 13, 2017, Arianna woke up from her coma. She started therapies to regain control of her motion and talking. Once well enough, she was transferred from the PICU unit down to pediatrics. As for Brent, he was in the ICU for a month-and-a-half before he was moved to a lower level in the hospital. He was doing better but still unconscious and needing twenty-four hour care. On February 7, 2017, Arianna was discharged from Dartmouth Hospital and transferred to Spaulding Rehabilitation Center in Charlestown, Massachusetts so she could get well enough to finally go home.

Arianna's progress was incredible, but Brent was still struggling to wake fully and overcome episodes of storming. Storming is what happens to people after they've had a brain injury, often times it is comes in episodes causing posturing or tightening of the whole body, high blood pressure spikes, anxiety, tachycardia as well as other symptoms.

> **Through it all, they never gave up and worked so hard to get to where they are today.**

The amount of trauma Brent and Arianna had to go through both physically and mentally can never fully be described. It was so sad to watch but also inspiring. Through it all, they never gave up and worked so hard to get to where they are today. It has been two years and counting since their car accident. Arianna is four years old and is doing better than ever. She loves swimming, running, learning and she's happy. Brent is 28 years old, improving more each day at his new rehab. Although he cannot walk and is still very disabled physically, his wheelchair gives him the independence to move around. He enjoys music, television and special visits from loved ones. Brent has spoken countless times since his accident but suffers from aphasia unfortunately, so it's a very rare occurrence.

He communicates with his eyes and expressions and always finds ways to show our mother or nurses what he wants or needs. He has a will to live and he doesn't give up! No matter what comes his way, illness or other obstacles, Brent never gives up. My only hope is that our family's story can bring hope to others who may have experienced this or may feel hopeless. Never give up on your loved ones and always be there for them no matter what journey they have ahead of them.

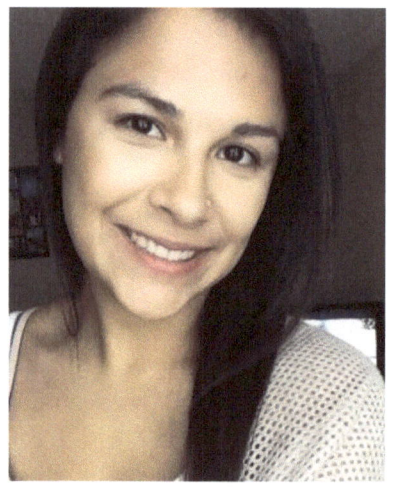

Meet Kiana Kay

Kiana Kay, a former Ophthalmic Technician is now a stay at home mother of one. When she is not outside exploring with her little one and significant other, she is at home teaching her daughter using the Montessori Method. She is the proud little sister of a very resilient traumatic brain injury survivor and spends most of her free time outdoors or going to the beaches of sunny Florida where she resides.

News & Views

We think that you'll agree – the April issue of HOPE Magazine was quite an inspirational issue. Brain injury has many facets and involves so much more than the survivor. As you've just read, moms, dads, siblings, children, parents – virtually all are affected.

Once brain injury becomes part of life, it takes the efforts of so many to help not only the survivor, but everyone else, to regain a new footing. It is very much a team effort in the truest sense. And so it is with HOPE Magazine. We provide the mechanism to help bring stories to the world, but our contributors are the real stars.

A couple of months ago we had an unimaginable conversation as story submissions slowed to crawl, and we wondered whether HOPE Magazine had effectively run its course. Everything has a beginning and an ending. It's the nature of all things. But we didn't throw in the towel easily and reached out to our contributing writers. The heroes that they are, they came to the rescue!

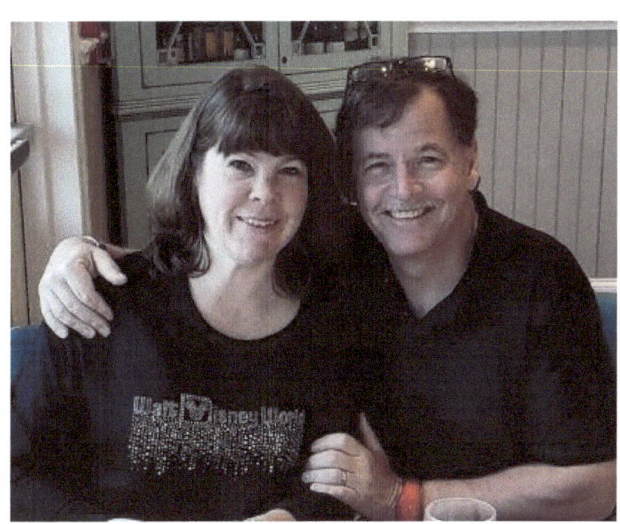

If you've come to appreciate all that HOPE Magazine has to offer, we are asking that you consider a story submission. You don't need to be an established writer. Some of our most compelling stories have come from the most unexpected contributors.

And so we circle back to you – the readers and writers who are part of our family of HOPE. Your words and stories have circled the globe, offering light in the darkest of places. We don't kid ourselves for a moment – you are Hope Magazine.

Peace,

~David & Sarah